MELANOMA CANCER COOKBOOK

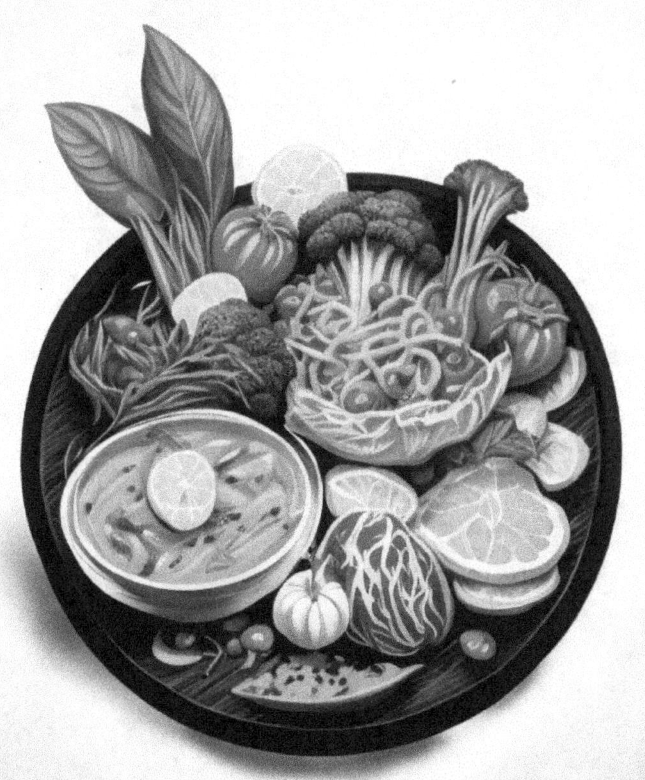

GET READY, LET'S FIGHT!

THIS BOOK BELONGS TO

Melanoma Cancer Cookbook

================================

Feeding Hope, Nurturing Health

Jetta Harlow Olson

Attribution: The resources utilized to design this cover were obtained from pexels.com.

ISBN: 9798857427859

Imprint: Independently Published

Disclaimer

This book's instructions, recommendations, or methods are not intended to replace professional medical guidance, diagnosis, or care. The information in this book is only meant to be used for educational purposes; it should not be used as a replacement for professional medical advice from a healthcare provider.

The authors and publisher of this book disclaim any responsibility for any negative effects or outcomes attributable to the use of the knowledge, suggestions, or methods offered in this book. Readers should speak with their doctor before beginning any new health or wellness program.

Despite the fact that the knowledge and research upon which the information in this book is based is up-to-date, medical procedures and recommendations may alter over time.

It is advised that readers seek out additional information and keep current with healthcare trends.

The authors' views are the only ones that are expressed in this book; they do not necessarily represent the publisher's views. The authors and publisher do not endorse or recommend any companies, items, or services that are mentioned in this book.

Despite making every effort to ensure the accuracy and comprehensiveness of the information in this book, the authors and publisher make no promises or representations of any kind, either explicitly or implicitly, regarding the information's suitability, reliability, or availability.

Any risks associated with relying on the information in this book are assumed by the reader.

Contents

1. Personal Motivation for the Cookbook

Creating a cookbook focused on melanoma cancer-friendly recipes is a deeply personal and meaningful endeavor. The motivation behind this cookbook stems from a desire to provide nourishing and flavorful options for individuals navigating the challenges of melanoma and its treatment journey. By sharing these recipes, you aim to empower those affected by melanoma with a valuable resource that not only supports their physical well-being but also uplifts their spirits during a challenging time.

Your personal motivation could be driven by various factors:

Empathy and Compassion: Your empathy for those impacted by melanoma fuels your dedication to offering recipes that are both nutritious and enjoyable. You understand the importance of maintaining a balanced diet to support the body's strength and resilience during treatment.

Culinary Creativity: Your passion for cooking and culinary creativity drives you to develop recipes that prove that health-conscious meals can be both delicious and visually appealing. Your goal is to demonstrate that flavorful options are within reach even when facing dietary restrictions.

Supportive Community: You aspire to create a sense of community and connection among individuals impacted by melanoma. Sharing recipes and meal ideas can foster a supportive environment where people can exchange tips, experiences, and encouragement.

Family or Personal Experience: If you or a loved one have personally experienced the challenges of melanoma, your cookbook can be an extension of your journey. It reflects your commitment to transforming adversity into an opportunity to help others facing similar struggles.

Positive Impact: Your aspiration to make a positive impact drives you to provide practical solutions that enhance the quality of life for melanoma patients and survivors. By addressing nutritional needs, you contribute to their overall well-being and outlook on their health journey.

Educational Advocacy: Through this cookbook, you seek to raise awareness about the role of nutrition in supporting cancer patients. You aim to educate both individuals directly impacted by melanoma and the broader community about the significance of a well-balanced diet.

Legacy of Hope: Your cookbook can serve as a legacy of hope and resilience. It symbolizes your commitment to spreading positivity and offering practical tools to empower individuals to take charge of their health.

Remember to infuse your personal motivations into the introduction or preface of the cookbook. By sharing your story and the driving forces behind this project, you can connect with your audience on a deeper level and inspire them to embrace the recipes with enthusiasm and appreciation.

Important Note: These recipes offer a variety of nutrient-rich ingredients and cater to different dietary preferences. Remember to tailor the portion sizes and ingredients to suit individual needs and dietary restrictions. Always consult with a healthcare professional before making significant changes to a patient's diet, especially for individuals undergoing cancer treatment.

2. Quinoa and Vegetable Salad

Ingredients:

- 1 cup cooked quinoa

- Mixed vegetables (bell peppers, cucumber, cherry tomatoes, red onion), chopped

- Fresh herbs (parsley, basil), chopped

- Olive oil and lemon juice for dressing

- Salt and pepper to taste

Instructions:

1. Cook quinoa according to package instructions and let it cool.

2. In a bowl, combine cooked quinoa, chopped vegetables, and fresh herbs.

3. Drizzle with olive oil and lemon juice, and season with salt and pepper.

4. Toss well and serve as a light and nutrient-rich salad.

3. Baked Salmon with Roasted Vegetables

Ingredients:

- Fresh salmon fillets

- Assorted vegetables (broccoli, carrots, zucchini), chopped

- Olive oil

- Garlic powder, paprika, salt, and pepper

Instructions:

1. Preheat the oven to 400°F (200°C).

2. Place salmon fillets on a baking sheet lined with parchment paper.

3. Toss chopped vegetables in olive oil, garlic powder, paprika, salt, and pepper.

4. Arrange vegetables around the salmon on the baking sheet.

5. Bake for about 15-20 minutes, or until the salmon is cooked and flakes easily with a fork.

6. Serve the salmon alongside the roasted vegetables.

4. Spinach and Berry Smoothie

Ingredients:

- Handful of spinach leaves

- Mixed berries (strawberries, blueberries, raspberries)

- Greek yogurt or dairy-free alternative

- Almond milk or other milk alternatives

- Honey or a touch of maple syrup (optional)

Instructions:

1. Blend spinach leaves, mixed berries, Greek yogurt, and almond milk until smooth.

2. Add honey or maple syrup for sweetness, if desired.

3. Pour into a glass and enjoy this nutrient-packed smoothie.

5. Chicken and Vegetable Stir-Fry

Ingredients:

- Boneless, skinless chicken breast, sliced

- Assorted vegetables (broccoli, bell peppers, snow peas), sliced

- Low-sodium soy sauce

- Fresh ginger and garlic, minced

- Olive oil

Instructions:

1. Heat olive oil in a skillet or wok over medium-high heat.

2. Add sliced chicken and cook until no longer pink. Remove from the skillet.

3. In the same skillet, add a bit more oil if needed and sauté minced ginger and garlic.

4. Add sliced vegetables and stir-fry until they're tender-crisp.

5. Return the cooked chicken to the skillet, add a splash of low-sodium soy sauce, and toss to combine.

6. Serve over brown rice or quinoa.

6. Chia Seed Pudding

Ingredients:

- Chia seeds

- Almond milk or other milk alternatives

- Fresh fruits (mango, berries) for topping

- Nuts or seeds for added crunch

Instructions:

1. Mix chia seeds and almond milk in a bowl. Use about 3-4 tablespoons of chia seeds for every cup of milk.

2. Stir well and let it sit in the refrigerator for a few hours or overnight until it thickens into a pudding-like consistency.

3. Serve with fresh fruits and nuts or seeds on top for added flavor and texture.

7. Roasted Beet and Walnut Salad

Ingredients:

- Roasted beets, sliced

- Mixed greens (spinach, arugula)

- Walnuts, chopped

- Goat cheese or feta cheese (optional)

- Balsamic vinaigrette dressing

Instructions:

1. Arrange mixed greens on a plate.

2. Top with roasted beet slices, chopped walnuts, and crumbled cheese, if using.

3. Drizzle with balsamic vinaigrette and enjoy this vibrant and nutrient-packed salad.

8. Lentil and Vegetable Soup

Ingredients:

- Green or brown lentils

- Assorted vegetables (carrots, celery, onion)

- Low-sodium vegetable broth

- Herbs and spices (thyme, rosemary, bay leaves)

- Olive oil

Instructions:

1. Heat olive oil in a large pot and sauté chopped vegetables until they soften.

2. Add lentils, herbs, and spices, and stir for a minute.

3. Pour in vegetable broth and bring to a boil. Reduce heat and let it simmer until lentils are tender.

4. Remove bay leaves before serving. This hearty soup is full of fiber and nutrients.

9. Grilled Veggie and Hummus Wrap

Ingredients:

- Whole-grain or gluten-free wrap
- Grilled vegetables (zucchini, eggplant, bell peppers)
- Hummus
- Fresh spinach or arugula

Instructions:

1. Spread a generous layer of hummus on the wrap.
2. Place grilled vegetables and fresh greens on top.
3. Roll up the wrap and cut it in half. It's a flavorful and satisfying meal.

10.Turmeric-Cauliflower Rice Stir-Fry

Ingredients:

- Cauliflower, grated or pulsed into rice-like texture
- Turmeric powder
- Mixed vegetables (peas, carrots, corn)
- Tofu or lean protein of choice, cubed
- Low-sodium soy sauce
- Sesame oil

Instructions:

1. In a skillet, heat sesame oil and sauté tofu until golden.
2. Add mixed vegetables and stir-fry until slightly tender.
3. Add cauliflower rice and turmeric powder, and stir well.
4. Drizzle with low-sodium soy sauce and continue cooking until heated through. It's a colorful and nutritious stir-fry.

11.Oatmeal with Mixed Berries and Almonds

Ingredients:

- Rolled oats

- Almond milk or other milk alternatives

- Mixed berries (blueberries, strawberries, raspberries)

- Sliced almonds

- Honey or maple syrup (optional)

Instructions:

1. Cook oats with almond milk according to package instructions.

2. Top with mixed berries, sliced almonds, and a drizzle of honey or maple syrup.

3. This wholesome breakfast is rich in fiber, antioxidants, and healthy fats.

12.Sweet Potato and Black Bean Bowl

Ingredients:

- Roasted sweet potatoes, diced
- Cooked black beans
- Quinoa or brown rice
- Avocado slices
- Salsa or pico de gallo

Instructions:

1. Assemble a bowl with quinoa or brown rice at the base.
2. Top with roasted sweet potatoes, black beans, avocado slices, and a spoonful of salsa.
3. This bowl is packed with fiber, protein, and healthy fats.

13.Ginger-Turmeric Carrot Soup

Ingredients:

- Carrots, chopped
- Onion, chopped
- Fresh ginger, grated
- Ground turmeric
- Low-sodium vegetable broth
- Coconut milk (light or full-fat)
- Fresh cilantro for garnish

Instructions:

1. In a pot, sauté chopped onion and grated ginger until fragrant.

2. Add chopped carrots and ground turmeric, and stir for a few minutes.

3. Pour in vegetable broth and bring to a simmer until carrots are tender.

4. Blend the mixture until smooth, then stir in coconut milk.

5. Garnish with fresh cilantro before serving.

14.Mediterranean Chickpea Salad

Ingredients:

- Canned chickpeas, drained and rinsed

- Cucumber, diced

- Cherry tomatoes, halved

- Red onion, finely chopped

- Kalamata olives, sliced

- Feta cheese (optional)

- Lemon vinaigrette dressing

Instructions:

1. In a large bowl, combine chickpeas, diced cucumber, halved cherry tomatoes, chopped red onion, and sliced olives.

2. Add crumbled feta cheese if using.

3. Drizzle with lemon vinaigrette and toss to combine.

15.Salmon and Avocado Sushi Bowl

Ingredients:

- Cooked sushi rice

- Cooked or grilled salmon, flaked

- Avocado slices

- Cucumber, julienned

- Nori seaweed, shredded

- Pickled ginger and wasabi (optional)

- Soy sauce or tamari (low-sodium)

Instructions:

1. Create a sushi bowl by layering cooked sushi rice with flaked salmon, avocado slices, julienned cucumber, and shredded nori seaweed.

2. Add pickled ginger and a touch of wasabi for extra flavor.

3. Serve with a side of low-sodium soy sauce or tamari.

16. Berry-Nut Parfait

Ingredients:

- Greek yogurt or dairy-free yogurt alternative

- Mixed berries (strawberries, blueberries, raspberries)

- Nuts and seeds (almonds, chia seeds)

- Honey or maple syrup (optional)

Instructions:

1. In a glass or bowl, layer Greek yogurt with mixed berries and a sprinkle of nuts and seeds.

2. Drizzle with honey or maple syrup if desired.

3. Repeat the layers and create a visually appealing and nutrient-rich parfait.

17.Broccoli and Almond Stir-Fry

Ingredients:

- Broccoli florets

- Sliced almonds

- Garlic, minced

- Low-sodium vegetable broth

- Lemon zest

- Crushed red pepper flakes (optional)

- Whole-wheat pasta or brown rice

Instructions:

1. Steam or blanch broccoli florets until tender-crisp.

2. In a skillet, sauté sliced almonds and minced garlic until fragrant.

3. Add steamed broccoli to the skillet along with a splash of low-sodium vegetable broth.

4. Sprinkle lemon zest and crushed red pepper flakes for a hint of heat.

5. Serve over whole-wheat pasta or brown rice.

18.Mango and Avocado Salad

Ingredients:

- Ripe mango, diced

- Avocado, diced

- Mixed greens (spinach, arugula)

- Red onion, thinly sliced

- Chopped fresh mint

- Lime juice and zest

Instructions:

1. Combine diced mango and avocado with mixed greens in a bowl.

2. Add thinly sliced red onion and chopped fresh mint.

3. Drizzle with lime juice and zest for a refreshing and tropical salad.

19. Veggie and Brown Rice Bowl with Tahini Dressing

Ingredients:

- Cooked brown rice

- Assorted roasted vegetables (bell peppers, zucchini, eggplant)

- Chickpeas, drained and rinsed

- Tahini dressing (tahini, lemon juice, garlic, water)

- Fresh parsley or cilantro for garnish

Instructions:

1. Assemble a bowl with cooked brown rice as the base.

2. Top with roasted vegetables and chickpeas.

3. Drizzle with tahini dressing and garnish with fresh parsley or cilantro.

20. Coconut-Berry Chia Pudding

Ingredients:

- Chia seeds

- Coconut milk (light or full-fat)

- Mixed berries (blueberries, raspberries, blackberries)

- Unsweetened shredded coconut

Instructions:

1. Mix chia seeds with coconut milk in a bowl and let it sit to thicken.

2. Layer chia pudding with mixed berries in serving glasses or jars.

3. Sprinkle unsweetened shredded coconut on top for extra texture and flavor.

21.Spinach and Mushroom Frittata

Ingredients:

- Eggs or egg substitute
- Fresh spinach leaves
- Sliced mushrooms
- Onion, chopped
- Low-fat cheese (optional)
- Fresh herbs (thyme, parsley)
- Salt and pepper

Instructions:

1. In a skillet, sauté chopped onion and sliced mushrooms until soft.
2. Add fresh spinach leaves and stir until wilted.
3. Beat eggs with fresh herbs, salt, and pepper, then pour over the vegetable mixture.
4. Cook on low heat until the edges set, then transfer to a preheated oven and bake until the center is cooked through.
5. Sprinkle with low-fat cheese if using and let it melt before serving.

22.Blueberry-Walnut Oat Bars

Ingredients:

- Rolled oats

- Almond flour

- Chopped walnuts

- Fresh blueberries

- Maple syrup

- Coconut oil

Instructions:

1. Mix rolled oats, almond flour, and chopped walnuts in a bowl.

2. In a separate bowl, combine melted coconut oil and maple syrup.

3. Combine wet and dry ingredients and fold in fresh blueberries.

4. Press the mixture into a baking pan and bake until golden and set.

5. Once cooled, cut into bars for a nutritious snack.

23. Cucumber and Dill Greek Yogurt Dip

Ingredients:

- Greek yogurt or dairy-free yogurt

- Cucumber, finely grated and squeezed to remove excess moisture

- Fresh dill, chopped

- Lemon juice and zest

- Garlic powder

- Salt and pepper

Instructions:

1. Mix Greek yogurt, finely grated cucumber, chopped dill, lemon juice, and zest.

2. Add a dash of garlic powder, salt, and pepper for flavor.

3. Serve as a dip with sliced vegetables or whole-grain crackers.

24.Roasted Brussels Sprouts with Pomegranate Seeds

Ingredients:

- Brussels sprouts, trimmed and halved

- Olive oil

- Pomegranate seeds

- Balsamic vinegar reduction (optional)

- Chopped toasted pecans (optional)

Instructions:

1. Toss halved Brussels sprouts in olive oil and roast until crispy.

2. Sprinkle with pomegranate seeds for a burst of color and antioxidants.

3. Drizzle with balsamic vinegar reduction and top with chopped toasted pecans, if desired.

25.Lentil and Vegetable Stuffed Bell Peppers

Ingredients:

- Bell peppers, halved and seeds removed

- Cooked green or brown lentils

- Mixed vegetables (carrots, zucchini, corn)

- Cooked quinoa or brown rice

- Tomato sauce

- Italian seasoning blend

Instructions:

1. Preheat the oven to 375°F (190°C).

2. Mix cooked lentils, mixed vegetables, cooked quinoa or brown rice, and a touch of tomato sauce.

3. Season with Italian seasoning blend.

4. Stuff the mixture into halved bell peppers and bake until the peppers are tender.

26.Almond-Crusted Baked Chicken

Ingredients:

- Boneless, skinless chicken breasts

- Whole wheat breadcrumbs or almond meal

- Crushed almonds

- Dijon mustard

- Fresh lemon juice

- Olive oil

- Salt and pepper

Instructions:

1. Preheat the oven to 400°F (200°C).

2. In a bowl, mix whole wheat breadcrumbs or almond meal with crushed almonds.

3. In a separate bowl, combine Dijon mustard, fresh lemon juice, olive oil, salt, and pepper.

4. Dip each chicken breast in the mustard mixture, then coat with the almond breadcrumb mixture.

5. Place the coated chicken breasts on a baking sheet and bake until golden and cooked through.

27.Grilled Veggie and Quinoa Stuffed Portobello Mushrooms

Ingredients:

- Portobello mushrooms, stems removed

- Assorted grilled vegetables (eggplant, bell peppers, zucchini)

- Cooked quinoa

- Fresh basil, chopped

- Balsamic glaze (reduction)

Instructions:

1. Preheat the grill.

2. Brush portobello mushrooms with olive oil and grill until tender.

3. Fill each mushroom with grilled vegetables and cooked quinoa.

4. Garnish with chopped fresh basil and drizzle with balsamic glaze.

28.Orange-Ginger Salmon Skewers

Ingredients:

- Salmon fillets, cut into cubes

- Fresh orange juice and zest

- Grated ginger

- Low-sodium soy sauce

- Honey or maple syrup

- Skewers (wooden or metal)

Instructions:

1. In a bowl, mix fresh orange juice and zest, grated ginger, low-sodium soy sauce, and a touch of honey or maple syrup.

2. Thread salmon cubes onto skewers and brush with the orange-ginger marinade.

3. Grill or bake the skewers until the salmon is cooked through and flakes easily.

29.Roasted Cauliflower and Chickpea Salad

Ingredients:

- Cauliflower florets

- Canned chickpeas, drained and rinsed

- Mixed greens (kale, spinach)

- Red onion, thinly sliced

- Tahini dressing (tahini, lemon juice, water)

- Chopped fresh parsley

Instructions:

1. Toss cauliflower florets and chickpeas in olive oil and roast until golden.

2. Combine roasted cauliflower and chickpeas with mixed greens and thinly sliced red onion.

3. Drizzle with tahini dressing and garnish with chopped fresh parsley.

30. Berry Quinoa Breakfast Bowl

Ingredients:

- Cooked quinoa

- Mixed berries (strawberries, blueberries, raspberries)

- Chopped nuts (almonds, walnuts)

- Unsweetened coconut flakes

- Greek yogurt or dairy-free yogurt

Instructions:

1. Assemble a bowl with cooked quinoa as the base.

2. Top with mixed berries, chopped nuts, and unsweetened coconut flakes.

3. Add a dollop of Greek yogurt or dairy-free yogurt for creaminess.

31.Pumpkin and Carrot Soup with Turmeric

Ingredients:

- Pumpkin puree (canned or homemade)

- Carrots, chopped

- Onion, chopped

- Ground turmeric

- Low-sodium vegetable broth

- Coconut milk (light or full-fat)

- Fresh cilantro or parsley for garnish

Instructions:

1. In a pot, sauté chopped onion and carrots until softened.

2. Add pumpkin puree and ground turmeric, stirring for a few minutes.

3. Pour in vegetable broth and bring to a simmer until the carrots are tender.

4. Blend the mixture until smooth and stir in coconut milk.

5. Garnish with fresh cilantro or parsley before serving.

32. Rainbow Quinoa Salad

Ingredients:

- Cooked tri-color quinoa

- Baby spinach

- Shredded purple cabbage

- Shredded carrots

- Diced red bell pepper

- Chopped cucumber

- Sunflower seeds

- Lemon-tahini dressing (tahini, lemon juice, water, garlic)

Instructions:

1. In a large bowl, combine cooked quinoa, baby spinach, shredded purple cabbage, shredded carrots, diced red bell pepper, and chopped cucumber.

2. Toss with sunflower seeds and drizzle with lemon-tahini dressing.

33. Turmeric-Ginger Smoothie

Ingredients:

- Fresh or frozen banana

- Pineapple chunks

- Fresh ginger, grated

- Ground turmeric

- Unsweetened almond milk or other milk alternatives

- Chia seeds or flax seeds (optional)

Instructions:

1. Blend banana, pineapple, grated ginger, ground turmeric, and almond milk until smooth.

2. Add chia seeds or flax seeds for added fiber and nutrients.

34.Mediterranean Tuna Salad

Ingredients:

- Canned tuna, drained

- Cherry tomatoes, halved

- Cucumber, diced

- Kalamata olives, sliced

- Red onion, finely chopped

- Feta cheese (optional)

- Olive oil and lemon juice dressing

- Fresh oregano or basil leaves for garnish

Instructions:

1. In a bowl, combine canned tuna, cherry tomatoes, diced cucumber, sliced olives, and finely chopped red onion.

2. Add crumbled feta cheese if desired.

3. Drizzle with olive oil and lemon juice dressing and garnish with fresh oregano or basil leaves.

35.Herbed Quinoa-Stuffed Acorn Squash

Ingredients:

- Acorn squash, halved and seeds removed
- Cooked quinoa
- Chopped fresh herbs (rosemary, thyme, parsley)
- Chopped nuts (pecans, almonds)
- Dried cranberries or raisins
- Olive oil

Instructions:

1. Preheat the oven to 375°F (190°C).
2. Brush acorn squash halves with olive oil and roast until tender.
3. Mix cooked quinoa with chopped herbs, chopped nuts, and dried cranberries or raisins.
4. Fill each acorn squash half with the quinoa mixture.

36.Green Pea and Mint Soup

Ingredients:

- Frozen green peas
- Fresh mint leaves
- Onion, chopped
- Low-sodium vegetable broth
- Lemon zest and juice
- Greek yogurt or dairy-free yogurt (optional)

Instructions:

1. In a pot, sauté chopped onion until translucent.
2. Add frozen green peas and fresh mint leaves, and stir briefly.
3. Pour in low-sodium vegetable broth and bring to a simmer.
4. Blend the mixture until smooth, then stir in lemon zest and juice.
5. Serve with a dollop of Greek yogurt or dairy-free yogurt, if desired.

37.Walnut-Crusted Chicken Tenders

Ingredients:

- Chicken tenders or boneless, skinless chicken breasts

- Whole wheat breadcrumbs or almond meal

- Chopped walnuts

- Dijon mustard

- Fresh lemon juice

- Olive oil

- Salt and pepper

Instructions:

1. Preheat the oven to 400°F (200°C).

2. In a bowl, mix whole wheat breadcrumbs or almond meal with chopped walnuts.

3. In another bowl, combine Dijon mustard, fresh lemon juice, olive oil, salt, and pepper.

4. Dip each chicken tender into the mustard mixture, then coat with the walnut breadcrumb mixture.

5. Place the coated chicken tenders on a baking sheet and bake until cooked through.

38.Mediterranean Quinoa-Stuffed Peppers

Ingredients:

- Bell peppers, halved and seeds removed

- Cooked quinoa

- Chopped tomatoes

- Chopped cucumber

- Chopped fresh parsley

- Crumbled feta cheese (optional)

- Lemon-oregano vinaigrette (olive oil, lemon juice, dried oregano)

Instructions:

1. Preheat the oven to 375°F (190°C).

2. Fill halved bell peppers with a mixture of cooked quinoa, chopped tomatoes, chopped cucumber, and chopped fresh parsley.

3. Add crumbled feta cheese if desired.

4. Drizzle with lemon-oregano vinaigrette before serving.

39.Mango-Coconut Chia Popsicles

Ingredients:

- Ripe mango, peeled and diced
- Coconut milk (light or full-fat)
- Chia seeds
- Honey or maple syrup (optional)

Instructions:

1. Blend diced mango with coconut milk until smooth.
2. Stir in chia seeds and let the mixture sit until it thickens.
3. Sweeten with honey or maple syrup if desired.
4. Pour the mixture into popsicle molds and freeze until solid.

40.Spinach and Mushroom Omelette

Ingredients:

- Eggs or egg substitute

- Fresh spinach leaves

- Sliced mushrooms

- Chopped onion

- Low-fat cheese (optional)

- Fresh herbs (chives, parsley)

- Salt and pepper

Instructions:

1. In a skillet, sauté chopped onion and sliced mushrooms until tender.

2. Add fresh spinach leaves and stir until wilted.

3. Beat eggs with fresh herbs, salt, and pepper, then pour over the vegetable mixture.

4. Cook until the omelette sets, then fold in half.

5. Add low-fat cheese if using and let it melt before serving.

41.Apple and Walnut Salad with Yogurt Dressing

Ingredients:

- Mixed greens (romaine, spinach, arugula)

- Sliced apples

- Chopped walnuts

- Dried cranberries

- Greek yogurt or dairy-free yogurt

- Honey or maple syrup

- Lemon juice

Instructions:

1. Combine mixed greens, sliced apples, chopped walnuts, and dried cranberries in a bowl.

2. Mix Greek yogurt with honey or maple syrup and a splash of lemon juice to make the dressing.

3. Drizzle the yogurt dressing over the salad before serving.

42.Butternut Squash and Apple Soup

Ingredients:

- Butternut squash, peeled and diced

- Apples, peeled, cored, and diced

- Onion, chopped

- Low-sodium vegetable broth

- Ground cinnamon

- Nutmeg

- Coconut milk (light or full-fat)

- Chopped fresh sage for garnish

Instructions:

1. In a pot, sauté chopped onion until translucent.

2. Add diced butternut squash and apples, and cook for a few minutes.

3. Pour in low-sodium vegetable broth and add ground cinnamon and nutmeg to taste.

4. Simmer until the squash and apples are tender, then blend until smooth.

5. Stir in coconut milk and heat through. Garnish with chopped fresh sage.

43.Avocado and Chickpea Lettuce Wraps

Ingredients:

- Romaine or butter lettuce leaves
- Mashed avocado
- Cooked chickpeas, mashed or chopped
- Diced cucumber
- Diced red bell pepper
- Lemon juice
- Fresh cilantro or parsley for garnish

Instructions:

1. Lay out lettuce leaves as wraps.
2. Spread mashed avocado onto each leaf, then add mashed or chopped chickpeas.
3. Top with diced cucumber and red bell pepper.
4. Drizzle with lemon juice and garnish with fresh cilantro or parsley.

44.Herbed Lemon Salmon with Asparagus

Ingredients:

- Salmon fillets

- Fresh lemon juice and zest

- Chopped fresh herbs (dill, parsley, thyme)

- Asparagus spears

- Olive oil

- Salt and pepper

Instructions:

1. Preheat the oven to 400°F (200°C).

2. Place salmon fillets on a baking sheet lined with parchment paper.

3. Mix fresh lemon juice, lemon zest, and chopped herbs.

4. Brush the mixture over the salmon fillets.

5. Toss asparagus spears with olive oil, salt, and pepper, and arrange them on the baking sheet.

6. Bake until the salmon is cooked and flakes easily, and the asparagus is tender.

45.Almond-Berry Overnight Oats

Ingredients:

- Rolled oats

- Almond milk or other milk alternatives

- Mixed berries (blueberries, strawberries, raspberries)

- Chopped almonds

- Honey or maple syrup (optional)

Instructions:

1. In a jar, combine rolled oats, almond milk, mixed berries, and chopped almonds.

2. Sweeten with honey or maple syrup if desired.

3. Refrigerate overnight for a ready-to-eat nutritious breakfast.

46.Cauliflower and Broccoli Rice Stir-Fry

Ingredients:

- Cauliflower florets, pulsed into rice-like texture
- Broccoli florets, chopped
- Sliced carrots
- Snow peas or snap peas
- Low-sodium soy sauce or tamari
- Garlic and ginger, minced
- Sesame oil

Instructions:

1. Heat sesame oil in a skillet and sauté minced garlic and ginger until fragrant.
2. Add chopped vegetables and stir-fry until tender-crisp.
3. Stir in cauliflower rice and broccoli rice.
4. Drizzle with low-sodium soy sauce or tamari and continue to stir-fry until heated through.

47.Brown Rice and Edamame Salad

Ingredients:

- Cooked brown rice
- Steamed edamame
- Shredded carrots
- Sliced radishes
- Chopped green onions
- Sesame seeds
- Rice vinegar and sesame oil dressing

Instructions:

1. Combine cooked brown rice, steamed edamame, shredded carrots, sliced radishes, and chopped green onions in a bowl.

2. Sprinkle with sesame seeds and drizzle with rice vinegar and sesame oil dressing.

48.Lemon-Herb Grilled Shrimp Skewers

Ingredients:

- Shrimp, peeled and deveined

- Lemon zest and juice

- Chopped fresh herbs (parsley, basil, thyme)

- Garlic, minced

- Olive oil

- Salt and pepper

Instructions:

1. In a bowl, mix lemon zest, lemon juice, chopped herbs, minced garlic, olive oil, salt, and pepper.

2. Thread shrimp onto skewers and brush with the lemon-herb marinade.

3. Grill or cook until the shrimp are opaque and cooked through.

49. Berry Chia Jam

Ingredients:

- Mixed berries (strawberries, blueberries, raspberries)

- Chia seeds

- Lemon juice

- Honey or maple syrup (optional)

Instructions:

1. Blend mixed berries with lemon juice until smooth.

2. Stir in chia seeds and sweeten with honey or maple syrup if desired.

3. Allow the mixture to sit until it thickens, then refrigerate as a healthy jam alternative.

50.Mediterranean Roasted Eggplant Dip (Baba Ganoush)

Ingredients:

- Eggplant
- Lemon juice
- Tahini
- Garlic, minced
- Olive oil
- Ground cumin
- Chopped fresh parsley
- Whole wheat pita or vegetable sticks for dipping

Instructions:

1. Roast or grill the eggplant until the skin is charred and the flesh is soft.

2. Scoop out the flesh and blend with lemon juice, tahini, minced garlic, olive oil, and ground cumin until smooth.

3. Garnish with chopped fresh parsley and serve with whole wheat pita or vegetable sticks.

51.Mixed Berry Parfait with Nut Granola

Ingredients:

- Greek yogurt or dairy-free yogurt

- Mixed berries (blueberries, strawberries, raspberries)

- Nut granola (almonds, walnuts, rolled oats)

- Honey or maple syrup (optional)

Instructions:

1. Layer Greek yogurt with mixed berries in serving glasses or bowls.

2. Sprinkle nut granola on top for added crunch and flavor.

3. Sweeten with honey or maple syrup if desired.

52.Mediterranean Chickpea and Quinoa Salad

Ingredients:

- Cooked quinoa
- Cooked chickpeas
- Diced cucumber
- Cherry tomatoes, halved
- Chopped red onion
- Chopped fresh parsley
- Feta cheese (optional)
- Lemon-oregano vinaigrette (olive oil, lemon juice, dried oregano)

Instructions:

1. Combine cooked quinoa, cooked chickpeas, diced cucumber, cherry tomatoes, chopped red onion, and chopped fresh parsley in a bowl.

2. Add crumbled feta cheese if desired.

3. Drizzle with lemon-oregano vinaigrette and toss to combine.

53.Ginger-Infused Carrot Smoothie

Ingredients:

- Carrots, chopped

- Fresh ginger, grated

- Greek yogurt or dairy-free yogurt

- Almond milk or other milk alternatives

- Honey or maple syrup (optional)

Instructions:

1. Blend chopped carrots, grated ginger, Greek yogurt, and almond milk until smooth.

2. Sweeten with honey or maple syrup if desired.

3. This vibrant smoothie is packed with nutrients and antioxidants.

54.Quinoa-Stuffed Bell Peppers with Turkey

Ingredients:

- Bell peppers, halved and seeds removed

- Cooked quinoa

- Lean ground turkey

- Chopped tomatoes

- Chopped fresh herbs (parsley, basil)

- Olive oil

- Garlic powder, onion powder, paprika

- Low-sodium tomato sauce

Instructions:

1. Preheat the oven to 375°F (190°C).

2. Brown lean ground turkey in a skillet with olive oil and seasonings.

3. Mix cooked quinoa, browned turkey, chopped tomatoes, and chopped fresh herbs in a bowl.

4. Stuff bell pepper halves with the quinoa-turkey mixture.

5. Top with a drizzle of low-sodium tomato sauce and bake until peppers are tender.

55.Zucchini Noodles with Pesto

Ingredients:

- Zucchini, spiralized into noodles

- Fresh basil leaves

- Pine nuts

- Grated Parmesan cheese (optional)

- Garlic, minced

- Olive oil

- Lemon juice

Instructions:

1. Blend fresh basil leaves, pine nuts, grated Parmesan cheese (if using), minced garlic, olive oil, and lemon juice to make the pesto.

2. Toss zucchini noodles with the pesto for a refreshing and low-carb meal.

56.Roasted Sweet Potato and Kale Salad

Ingredients:

- Roasted sweet potatoes, diced

- Chopped kale leaves

- Toasted pumpkin seeds

- Dried cranberries

- Balsamic vinaigrette dressing

Instructions:

1. Arrange chopped kale leaves on a plate.

2. Top with roasted sweet potatoes, toasted pumpkin seeds, and dried cranberries.

3. Drizzle with balsamic vinaigrette for a flavorful and nutrient-rich salad.

57.Lemon-Dill Grilled Chicken Salad

Ingredients:

- Grilled chicken breast, sliced

- Mixed greens (arugula, spinach)

- Sliced cucumber

- Cherry tomatoes, halved

- Sliced red onion

- Chopped fresh dill

- Lemon vinaigrette dressing

Instructions:

1. Arrange mixed greens on a plate.

2. Top with sliced grilled chicken, sliced cucumber, halved cherry tomatoes, and sliced red onion.

3. Sprinkle with chopped fresh dill and drizzle with lemon vinaigrette.

58.Quinoa and Black Bean Stuffed Acorn Squash

Ingredients:

- Acorn squash, halved and seeds removed

- Cooked quinoa

- Cooked black beans

- Diced bell peppers (red, yellow, or orange)

- Chopped fresh cilantro

- Lime juice

- Ground cumin

Instructions:

1. Preheat the oven to 375°F (190°C).

2. Fill each acorn squash half with a mixture of cooked quinoa, cooked black beans, diced bell peppers, chopped fresh cilantro, lime juice, and ground cumin.

3. Bake until the squash is tender and the filling is heated through.

59.Blueberry-Almond Chia Seed Pudding

Ingredients:

- Chia seeds

- Almond milk or other milk alternatives

- Fresh blueberries

- Chopped almonds

- Vanilla extract

- Honey or maple syrup (optional)

Instructions:

1. Mix chia seeds with almond milk and vanilla extract in a bowl.

2. Layer chia seed pudding with fresh blueberries and chopped almonds.

3. Sweeten with honey or maple syrup if desired.

60.Cauliflower and White Bean Mash

Ingredients:

- Cauliflower florets

- Cooked white beans

- Garlic, minced

- Olive oil

- Fresh lemon juice

- Chopped fresh parsley

- Salt and pepper

Instructions:

1. Steam or boil cauliflower florets until tender.

2. In a food processor, blend cooked cauliflower, white beans, minced garlic, olive oil, and fresh lemon juice until smooth.

3. Season with chopped fresh parsley, salt, and pepper.

61.Chocolate-Banana Protein Smoothie

Ingredients:

- Ripe banana

- Unsweetened cocoa powder

- Greek yogurt or dairy-free yogurt

- Almond milk or other milk alternatives

- Nut butter (almond, peanut, or sunflower)

- Protein powder (plant-based)

- Ice cubes

Instructions:

1. Blend ripe banana, unsweetened cocoa powder, Greek yogurt, almond milk, nut butter, protein powder, and ice cubes until creamy.

2. This smoothie provides a tasty and protein-rich snack.

62.Cucumber and Avocado Gazpacho

Ingredients:

- Cucumbers, peeled and diced

- Ripe avocado, peeled and diced

- Green bell pepper, diced

- Red onion, chopped

- Fresh cilantro or parsley, chopped

- Low-sodium vegetable broth

- Lemon juice

- Salt and pepper

Instructions:

1. In a blender, combine diced cucumbers, diced avocado, diced green bell pepper, chopped red onion, and fresh cilantro or parsley.

2. Add low-sodium vegetable broth and a splash of lemon juice.

3. Blend until smooth and season with salt and pepper.

4. Serve chilled for a refreshing and light soup.

63.Quinoa-Stuffed Mushrooms

Ingredients:

- Portobello mushrooms, stems removed
- Cooked quinoa
- Chopped spinach
- Diced tomatoes
- Minced garlic
- Olive oil
- Grated Parmesan cheese (optional)
- Fresh basil leaves for garnish

Instructions:

1. Preheat the oven to 375°F (190°C).
2. Brush portobello mushrooms with olive oil and place them on a baking sheet.
3. In a bowl, mix cooked quinoa, chopped spinach, diced tomatoes, and minced garlic.
4. Fill each mushroom cap with the quinoa mixture.
5. Top with grated Parmesan cheese (if using) and bake until mushrooms are tender.
6. Garnish with fresh basil leaves before serving.

64.Grilled Tofu and Vegetable Skewers

Ingredients:

- Firm tofu, cubed

- Assorted vegetables (bell peppers, zucchini, cherry tomatoes, red onion)

- Marinade: Olive oil, lemon juice, garlic, dried herbs (oregano, thyme)

- Skewers (wooden or metal)

Instructions:

1. Mix olive oil, lemon juice, minced garlic, and dried herbs to make the marinade.

2. Thread cubed tofu and chopped vegetables onto skewers.

3. Brush with the marinade and grill until tofu is lightly browned and vegetables are tender.

65.Mixed Berry Chia Smoothie Bowl

Ingredients:

- Mixed berries (blueberries, raspberries, strawberries)

- Chia seeds

- Greek yogurt or dairy-free yogurt

- Almond milk or other milk alternatives

- Toppings: Sliced almonds, shredded coconut, granola

Instructions:

1. Blend mixed berries, chia seeds, Greek yogurt, and almond milk until smooth.

2. Pour the smoothie into a bowl.

3. Top with sliced almonds, shredded coconut, and granola for added texture and flavor.

66.Broccoli and Quinoa Stir-Fry

Ingredients:

- Broccoli florets

- Cooked quinoa

- Sliced bell peppers

- Sliced carrots

- Low-sodium soy sauce or tamari

- Ginger, minced

- Garlic, minced

- Sesame oil

Instructions:

1. Heat sesame oil in a skillet and sauté minced ginger and garlic until fragrant.

2. Add sliced bell peppers and sliced carrots and stir-fry until crisp-tender.

3. Stir in broccoli florets and cooked quinoa.

4. Drizzle with low-sodium soy sauce or tamari and continue to stir-fry until heated through.

67.Mediterranean Lentil Salad

Ingredients:

- Cooked green or brown lentils
- Chopped cucumber
- Diced red bell pepper
- Chopped Kalamata olives
- Chopped red onion
- Chopped fresh parsley
- Feta cheese (optional)
- Lemon-tahini dressing (tahini, lemon juice, water)

Instructions:

1. Combine cooked lentils, chopped cucumber, diced red bell pepper, chopped Kalamata olives, chopped red onion, and chopped fresh parsley in a bowl.

2. Add crumbled feta cheese if desired.

3. Drizzle with lemon-tahini dressing and toss to coat.

68.Almond Butter and Banana Overnight Oats

Ingredients:

- Rolled oats

- Almond butter

- Sliced ripe banana

- Almond milk or other milk alternatives

- Chia seeds

- Cinnamon

- Honey or maple syrup (optional)

Instructions:

1. In a jar, layer rolled oats, almond butter, sliced ripe banana, and chia seeds.

2. Add a dash of cinnamon and drizzle with honey or maple syrup if desired.

3. Pour almond milk over the layers and refrigerate overnight.

69.Roasted Beet and Orange Salad

Ingredients:

- Roasted beets, sliced

- Orange segments

- Mixed greens (arugula, spinach)

- Sliced red onion

- Chopped walnuts

- Orange vinaigrette dressing

Instructions:

1. Arrange mixed greens on a plate.

2. Top with sliced roasted beets, orange segments, sliced red onion, and chopped walnuts.

3. Drizzle with orange vinaigrette for a colorful and flavorful salad.

70.Spaghetti Squash with Marinara Sauce

Ingredients:

- Spaghetti squash, cooked and strands separated

- Homemade or low-sodium store-bought marinara sauce

- Chopped fresh basil

- Grated Parmesan cheese (optional)

- Red pepper flakes (optional)

Instructions:

1. Mix cooked spaghetti squash strands with marinara sauce.

2. Heat the mixture until warm.

3. Stir in chopped fresh basil and grated Parmesan cheese if using.

4. Serve with a sprinkle of red pepper flakes for added heat.

71.Berry-Walnut Breakfast Parfait

Ingredients:

- Greek yogurt or dairy-free yogurt

- Mixed berries (blueberries, raspberries, strawberries)

- Chopped walnuts

- Honey or maple syrup (optional)

Instructions:

1. In a glass or bowl, layer Greek yogurt with mixed berries and chopped walnuts.

2. Drizzle with honey or maple syrup if desired.

3. Repeat the layers and enjoy a wholesome breakfast parfait.

72.Pumpkin and Lentil Soup

Ingredients:

- Pumpkin puree (canned or homemade)
- Cooked green or brown lentils
- Low-sodium vegetable broth
- Onion, chopped
- Garlic, minced
- Ground turmeric
- Ground cumin
- Coconut milk (light or full-fat)
- Chopped fresh cilantro

Instructions:

1. In a pot, sauté chopped onion and minced garlic until softened.

2. Add pumpkin puree, cooked lentils, ground turmeric, and ground cumin.

3. Pour in low-sodium vegetable broth and simmer.

4. Blend the mixture until smooth, then stir in coconut milk.

5. Garnish with chopped fresh cilantro before serving.

73. Spinach and Mushroom Stuffed Chicken Breast

Ingredients:

- Chicken breasts, boneless and skinless
- Chopped spinach
- Sliced mushrooms
- Minced garlic
- Low-fat mozzarella cheese (optional)
- Olive oil
- Lemon zest
- Salt and pepper

Instructions:

1. Preheat the oven to 375°F (190°C).
2. In a skillet, sauté chopped spinach, sliced mushrooms, and minced garlic until cooked.
3. Butterfly the chicken breasts and stuff with the spinach and mushroom mixture.
4. Add low-fat mozzarella cheese if using.
5. Secure the chicken breasts with toothpicks, brush with olive oil, and sprinkle with lemon zest, salt, and pepper.

6. Bake until the chicken is cooked through and the cheese is melted.

74.Quinoa and Black Bean Burger

Ingredients:

- Cooked quinoa

- Cooked black beans

- Rolled oats

- Chopped bell peppers

- Chopped onion

- Ground cumin

- Smoked paprika

- Garlic powder

- Egg or flaxseed egg (for binding)

- Whole wheat burger buns or lettuce wraps

Instructions:

1. In a food processor, blend cooked quinoa, cooked black beans, rolled oats, chopped bell peppers, chopped onion, ground cumin, smoked paprika, and garlic powder.

2. Transfer the mixture to a bowl and stir in an egg or flaxseed egg for binding.

3. Form patties and cook on a skillet or grill until browned and cooked through.

4. Serve on whole wheat burger buns or lettuce wraps.

75.Berry Quinoa Parfait

Ingredients:

- Cooked quinoa

- Mixed berries (blueberries, strawberries, raspberries)

- Low-fat Greek yogurt or dairy-free yogurt

- Chopped nuts (almonds, walnuts)

- Honey or maple syrup (optional)

Instructions:

1. In a glass or bowl, layer cooked quinoa, mixed berries, and low-fat Greek yogurt.

2. Top with chopped nuts and drizzle with honey or maple syrup if desired.

3. Repeat the layers for a satisfying and nutritious parfait.

76.Roasted Vegetable Frittata

Ingredients:

- Mixed roasted vegetables (bell peppers, zucchini, onion, cherry tomatoes)

- Eggs or egg substitute

- Low-fat cheese (optional)

- Chopped fresh herbs (basil, thyme)

- Salt and pepper

Instructions:

1. Preheat the oven to 375°F (190°C).

2. In a baking dish, spread mixed roasted vegetables.

3. In a bowl, whisk eggs with low-fat cheese, chopped fresh herbs, salt, and pepper.

4. Pour the egg mixture over the roasted vegetables.

5. Bake until the frittata is set and lightly browned.

77.Rainbow Quinoa-Stuffed Bell Peppers

Ingredients:

- Bell peppers, halved and seeds removed

- Cooked rainbow quinoa

- Cooked lean ground turkey or chicken

- Chopped spinach

- Diced tomatoes

- Minced garlic

- Low-sodium vegetable broth

- Fresh basil, chopped

- Grated Parmesan cheese (optional)

Instructions:

1. Preheat the oven to 375°F (190°C).

2. In a bowl, mix cooked rainbow quinoa, cooked lean ground turkey or chicken, chopped spinach, diced tomatoes, and minced garlic.

3. Fill each bell pepper half with the quinoa mixture.

4. Pour a splash of low-sodium vegetable broth into the baking dish.

5. Bake until the peppers are tender and the filling is heated through.

6. Garnish with chopped fresh basil and grated Parmesan cheese if desired.

78.Citrus-Kale Salad with Grilled Chicken

Ingredients:

- Grilled chicken breast, sliced

- Chopped kale leaves

- Orange segments

- Sliced almonds

- Dried cranberries

- Orange vinaigrette dressing

Instructions:

1. Massage chopped kale leaves to soften.

2. Arrange kale on a plate and top with sliced grilled chicken, orange segments, sliced almonds, and dried cranberries.

3. Drizzle with orange vinaigrette for a zesty salad.

79.Chia Seed and Berry Smoothie

Ingredients:

- Mixed berries (blueberries, strawberries, raspberries)

- Chia seeds

- Almond milk or other milk alternatives

- Greek yogurt or dairy-free yogurt

- Honey or maple syrup (optional)

Instructions:

1. Blend mixed berries, chia seeds, almond milk, and Greek yogurt until smooth.

2. Sweeten with honey or maple syrup if desired.

3. This smoothie provides a boost of fiber and antioxidants.

80.Spinach and Feta Stuffed Mushrooms

Ingredients:

- Large mushroom caps

- Chopped spinach

- Crumbled feta cheese

- Minced garlic

- Olive oil

- Fresh lemon juice

- Chopped fresh dill

- Salt and pepper

Instructions:

1. Preheat the oven to 375°F (190°C).

2. In a skillet, sauté chopped spinach and minced garlic in olive oil until wilted.

3. Stir in crumbled feta cheese, fresh lemon juice, chopped fresh dill, salt, and pepper.

4. Fill each mushroom cap with the spinach and feta mixture.

5. Bake until the mushrooms are tender and the filling is heated.

81.Oat-Banana Pancakes

Ingredients:

- Rolled oats

- Ripe bananas, mashed

- Eggs or egg substitute

- Cinnamon

- Vanilla extract

- Baking powder

- Fresh berries for topping

- Greek yogurt or dairy-free yogurt for topping

Instructions:

1. Blend rolled oats to make oat flour.

2. Mix oat flour with mashed bananas, eggs, cinnamon, vanilla extract, and baking powder to make a pancake batter.

3. Cook the batter in a non-stick skillet until golden brown on both sides.

4. Top with fresh berries and a dollop of Greek yogurt or dairy-free yogurt.

= THE END =

We appreciate you selecting this book! We hope your expectations were fulfilled or surpassed.

Please think about posting a review on social media if you liked our book. We value your opinion because it enables us to make improvements to our goods and services for future clients.

We want to thank you once more for your support and send our best to you.